P9-DFP-735

Other Hippocrates Books
by Brian R. & Anna Maria Clement

#1 Hippocrates Health Program:
A Proven Guide to Healthful Living
#2 Belief: All There is
#3 Children: The Ultimate Creation
#5 Relationships: Voyages Through Life

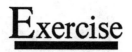

Exercise

Creating
Your
Persona

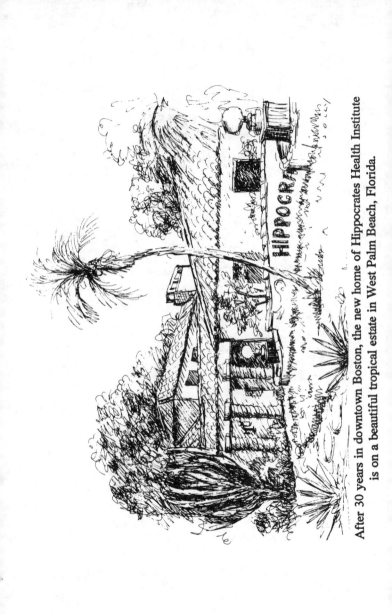

After 30 years in downtown Boston, the new home of Hippocrates Health Institute is on a beautiful tropical estate in West Palm Beach, Florida.

Exercise

Creating Your Persona

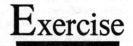

Brian R. Clement

Foreword by Sylvia Ortiz

A.M. Press   West Palm Beach, Florida

The medical and health procedures in this book are based on the training, personal experiences, and research of the author. Because each person and situation is unique, the author and publisher urge the reader to check with a qualified health professional before using any procedure where there is any question as to its appropriateness.

The publisher does not advocate the use of any particular diet and exercise program, but believes the information presented in this book should be available to the public.

Because there is always some risk involved, the author and publisher are not responsible for any adverse effects or consequences resulting from the use of any of the suggestions, preparations, or procedures in this book. Please do not use the book if you are unwilling to assume the risk. Feel free to consult a physician or other qualified health professional. It is a sign of wisdom, not cowardice, to seek a second or third opinion.

All rights reserved. No part of this publication may be reproduced, stored in a retrieval system, or transmitted in any form or by any means, electronic, mechanical, photocopying, or otherwise, without the prior written permission of the copyright owner. Published 1994

©1994 by Brian R. Clement

Printed in the United States of America

Library of Congress Cataloging-In-Publication Data
pending

Clement, Brian R.
   Exercise: Creating Your Persona
   ISBN 0-9622373-4-5

Cover and art illustrations by CAMF Productions
Typography and book design by Dianne Krause

*To every person
on the planet who
has the wisdom
to utilize our greatest gift
— the human body.*

Contents

Foreword

You are now on your way to having everything you really need to generate the most healthy and fit body you can. What is your reaction to what you just read? Did you start to regret the possibility? Only a fool would accept such a statement on absolute faith. But a wise person, free of deadly self-limitation would merely ask how.

Since the production of my videos "Rebound Exercise Video Series" and through my Healthy Cell presentations, I came in contact with an extraordinary arrary of dedicated people who are working to educate others on how to be truly healthy. Brian Clement stands out uniquely as a whole health leader. Recognize that total health is not a one-sided process that can be achieved with supplements and pills alone. Health is instead a balance of nutrition, exercise and beliefs.

Without a doubt Brian Clement has done it again, as he adds this book to his living health series. *Exercise: Creating Your Persona* is a hands-on approach which inspires all to get healthy through exercise. Young, old, overweight, fit or sick, no matter what the condition. Brian captures the true essence of exercise and its place in our lives. In this book, you will find out what a joy it is to move, laugh, run, play and have fun when you exercise. The vital information inside, the quality of your life really does depend on it. The choice is yours...and I hope you will make the right choice.

At this time, we must be acutely aware of our actions. The most significant action is that of exercise. Vigorous exercise not only builds a strong body but puts you in touch with yourself. In addition you will enjoy an increased lymph circulation and blood oxygen. A process that initiates the body's internal cleansing system, boosting one's energy level and preventing much human suffering

Inactivity has become this country's pastime. Unfortunately, this inactivity continues on its depressed cycle because people who are not in shape continue to deteriorate. With each day that passes, a person becomes more out of shape. In fact, people lose 10 percent of their fitness each day that they do not exercise.

The mere fact that we have 700 muscles affirms that our bodies were made for activity. Brian explains that exercise is more than simply moving the body. It is moving the mind and moving the life to a better and higher place. As you read through these pages, Brian's down-to-earth style will clearly show you how easy it is to embrace exercise and make it a joy and not a chore.

It is my hope that you will read this book as if your life depended on it...because as you read the vital information inside, the quality of your life really does depend on it. The choice is yours . . . and I hope you will make the right one.

Stay Fit and Healthy.

SYLVIA ORTIZ

National Rebound Authority
Author of *A Jump Ahead*

Preface

The most overlooked area of health is exercise. In recent years, exercise has become a faddish activity that is generally used either to reduce weight or to gain beauty. The essence of exercise is very seldom discussed or understood.

In the chapters that follow, I will explain the truth of exercise and how it is vital in one's experience and one's progress toward a happy and successful life. Exercise is not something we should think of as a chore, but something we should think of as a close friend — an effortless affair that brings us to higher levels of happiness and awareness.

No doubt that there was a time in my life when exercise was lacking, and now there is no doubt that I was missing a very large part of my health. There will never be a time in my life when exercise is not included, because without it, I feel there is no full life.

After reading this book, please start to utilize some of the thoughts and methods I suggest. Do not just intellectualize on the possibility at some futuristic date, but moreso engage the activity of the present moment.

Brian R. Clement

INTRODUCTION

Why is Exercise Important?

For some — the athletes, the aerobics instructors, the dieters and the fitness fanatics — that is a very obvious question. But for the rest of us, who are in relatively good shape, can still fit into our clothes and aren't drinking chocolate faux shakes for breakfast and lunch, the question is valid.

Exercise is more than bouncing around or lifting weights to look like muscle people. Exercise extends beyond the bone, muscle and ligaments and beyond the gym, track and pool. Exercise is mental. It is a thinking man's alternative: because before anyone can pick up a barbell or turn on that hated videotape, they already have to be in the top mental shape of their life. They already have to picture themselves well and healthy and trim and energized. But even before that, people who want to be physically fit have to understand that exercise transforms more than just the body. Exercise takes the mind to a new height.

How?

Exercise gives a person a daily challenge to better oneself. It opens up potential and a vast world of unknown strength and agility. It restores confidence and ability, and it makes the person feel better about themselves. A person has to understand the gift and wonder of exercise before he or she starts. Exercise is more than just a physical change. It is the beginning of a whole new realm of living.

As hokey as it may sound, exercise gives people a new lease on life. Imagine that simply using your body in the way that it was meant to be used could open so many doors and unleash so many opportunities. Astounding, isn't it? Too many people are caught in the deception that simply maintaining a body is enough; that if you are not horribly overweight or sick that exercise is an optional recreation. That is not true. Still others believe that three times a week for 30 minutes will sufficiently encompass all that one person needs to fulfill a lifetime of exercise. And some go as far as to adopt a mode of thinking that one form of exercise is all they'll ever need from childhood until death.

All of this is wrong. But it is not the fault of one man that this type of thinking came to be. It is society's instituted means of instilling skewed values of exercise; that it can be fit into a schedule, regimented like a drill school curriculum and carried out like direct orders: "You must exercise!"

Where's the incentive? Where's the knowledge? Where's the growth? Where's the joy?

It's a shame that most of us do not realize the higher, larger, more life-changing benefits of exercise: that it is a part of life in much the same way as eating, breathing and sleeping; that it should come as naturally as those three life processes; that exercise does not have to be confined to a gym or an aerobics class, done every other day from 6 a.m to 7 a.m.; that exercise is not our enemy, but our savior and that it is not reserved for the "healthy" people — that group of unbelievable human beings who eat the right amount of vegetables, drink eight glasses of water a day and sleep for eight hours. It is for everyone, right down to the woman who snacks on chips at 1 a.m. to the man who hasn't left his couch in 10 years.

Exercise is not a dirty word. When pursued correctly, it does not hurt. And when done consistently, it will not turn a man into a mammoth monster or a woman into a bulging, muscle-bound weight lifter. What it will do is make life more enjoyable. It will extend the wholesomeness of

4

your body and preserve its worth. It will energize and relax, strengthen and rejuvenate. It will expand the mind and release the spirit; knock down barriers and expose light.

Exercise can do all that. It's just a matter of believing it can, doing it, then sitting back and watching the results.

But believing that it can is a mental process. Remember, exercise is a thinking person's game. People have to believe the plane will fly before they board. She has to believe that the child will walk before she invests in shoes. He has to believe the car will start before he leaves for work. Just as practically, people have to believe exercise will make a difference in their lives before they do one jumping jack, run one lap or swim one length. Belief in the unknown has enlightened millions of people, put a man on the moon, and solved world diseases and plagues.

It is not beyond one's realm of comprehension simply to believe. Leave the doubts and misgivings where you found them — back years ago when exercise was a foreign concept — and get ready to introduce your mind to common sense, spirituality and the belief that exercise can change lives, improve bodies, increase confidence and propel a soul forward with the speed and grace of a gazelle.

Why is exercise important?

To live. Simply to live and live well.

CHAPTER 1

History Should Repeat Itself

Decades ago, exercise was not something that was decided to be accomplished. It was simply accomplished by living. There were no aerobics classes or psychedelic gyms. There were no videotapes or sports shops. No one yelled from a television screen the benefits of being on one fad diet versus another.

Exercise was not even about losing weight. As impossible as our society finds it to believe, exercise was a part of life, not something that was scheduled for after work or early in the morning. Exercise was a natural process, achieved through plain survival. Eating, growing, riding and working were all essential elements in a time when machines did not complete 90 percent of our work. Our grandmothers and grandfathers did not have the disadvantage of microwaves, blenders or even automobiles. Everything was done by hand and as a result everything was an exercise.

Just maintaining a home took washing the clothes with a scrubbing board and elbow grease, sweeping the floors with a broom made of straw, not a vacuum cleaner, cleaning dishes with a human washer, and drying sheets on a line in the sun: lifting and stretching, pulling and tugging; using the back, the arms, the chest and the legs. Cleaning a home was more than a collection of chemicals as they are now, that are sprayed and spritzed and foamed. It took effort and heart.

Making dinner was a process that started weeks prior with the planting of the seeds, after the soil was plowed and the animals were fed. Then the grains were crushed and mixed and beat and battered and baked. It is tiring to our generation of electrical gadgets and gimmicks to hear about the amount of work it took to just eat and remain clean.

It was that work that kept the hearts of our prior generations pumping with life and energy. Exercise was not discussed and analyzed, preached over and wished for. Exercise was the daily maintenance of living, and now with the advent of ever- increasing technology, the need to physically work for a living and exercise for sustenance has disappeared.

Even transportation has deprived this society of the motion it had when it was younger. Getting on horseback and going from home to the market was a daily, much anticipated journey. But the ride was more than fresh air and bright sun. The bouncing rhythm of the horses cleaned the lymphatic system, which helped the liver, the gall bladder and the overall body by decalcifying it.

It's hard to believe that motion helped clean the body. But it is true. What made a day full was what kept the pioneers of this country well. Diseases and viruses existed, but probably not to the degree they did when the Industrial Age began to boom; when machines began to do work that was reserved for back muscles and strong arms; when exercise started to become relegated to the back rooms of traditional fare and not part of a daily existence.

Now, as sad as it might seem, people do not work their bodies anymore. Just think about the list of modern gadgets that keep a man from moving, from working, from exercising: remote controls, vacuum cleaners, cars, buses, trains, video games, garbage disposals, portable phones and restaurants. Very few things today have to be sought because so much can be ordered, called in or delivered. In the United States alone, about 75 percent of the population have the means to pay other people for things. If one were to travel back 100 years, only 5 percent of the population had the money to do that.

The list continues: elevators, escalators, motorcycles and motorboats. Some would think exercise is not necessary anymore. Or is it?

Exercise in any form is always necessary. Most people recognize this loss in our lives and have gone through steps to replace the missing link of energy and motion.

Instead of horseback riding, today's exerciser invests in a mini-trampoline. The bouncing action imitates the rhythm of a horse to cleanse the lymphatic system. The bouncing also works against gravity to add in the cleansing process and build muscle.

During the 1984 Olympics, the American teams used rebounders with little sand bags in their hands which, when used against gravity, increased the weight of their bodies by 125 percent each. Working against gravity, muscles can be built inside a pool with resistant flaps and fins, moving against the pressure of the water in a very natural rhythm; working against gravity, using natural, rhythmic motions, pushing against the inherent barriers of nature. This is how the generations before us lived.

Just 100 years ago, about 92 percent of the population worked for food production. For the basic goals of securing a meal for their families and making a living by growing from the earth. While at work, they exposed themselves to sunlight, breathing fresh air, pushing their bodies to the maximum and growing because of it. Their immune systems benefited from the sun, their lungs benefited from the air and their bodies, their organs, and their lives benefited from the exercise.

Today, we call fitness what they called living. And it shouldn't be that way.

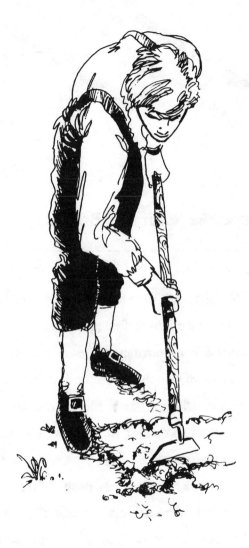

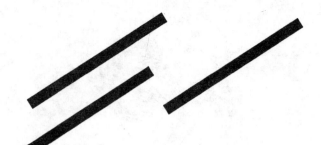

CHAPTER 2

Exercise: As Natural as Breathing

We shouldn't have to think about exercise. Exercise is not a bill to be fretted over or an outing to be planned. Unfortunately, these are sentiments to the droves of people who tune into any new celebrity appearing on the scene, telling society that exercise is something to solve weight gain, something that should be done 30 minutes a day for three days a week. It has been drilled into people's minds that exercise should not come naturally; should not be fun; should not be as common as taking a shower or going to work.

Instead of fitting in exercise, plan life with it. It is a mental challenge to imagine the world filled with people who did not bemoan exercising; who woke up in the morning without giving exercise a single thought. Why think about something that required no examination? Moving and using the body would be as natural as inhaling and exhaling, and very few individuals stop to contemplate their breathing. Should I stop breathing around 2 p.m. to give my lungs a rest? Will I breathe faster around 11 a.m., then slow down at 4 p.m.? Seems silly, doesn't it?

But that is how our generation approaches exercise, as something to be prepared, anticipated and dreaded. It makes no sense to dread something that can do nothing but help you expand your potential, fulfill your wishes and strengthen the heart, mind and soul.

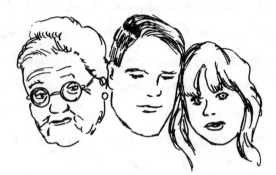

CHAPTER 3

Exercise: The Uncountable Benefits

Exercise is invigorating. It improves the physical appearance, tightening and toning, lifting and hardening. Beyond a strong body and an increased attractiveness, exercise creates circulation in the body, which detoxifies the tissues and builds muscle because circulation delivers oxygen to every part of the human system.

Oxygen is precious and vital because it feeds the mind, accelerates the muscles and increases the capacity to work and live. Even more, exercise delivers relaxation and self-esteem. When a person is fit, no longer do they worry about the fit of their clothes, their gait or their acceptance. With each day, confidence grows and a smile replaces the frown of insecurity and doubt.

Exercise should be viewed as fulfilling three goals:

The first goal should be to develop the body and stay fit. The more a person moves, the more free they become to move even further. Fitness comes from working against gravity, from increasing the tolerance for fatigue, from learning new skills and from testing limits and pushing against them. Greater fitness helps in all kinds of stressful situations, both physical and psychological.

The second goal should be to enjoy oneself and to have fun. The joy of movement comes from social contact, from competing and playing with friends, and from touching others. It comes from aesthetic experience, like moving gracefully and feeling the sun on your face. If a person is not having fun while they exercise, it's time to find some new games and rekindle the joy of childish play.

The third goal should be to nurture oneself and find fulfillment. Moving is a form of self-nurturance. Like eating and sleeping, it meets a basic human need. If people love their dogs, they walk them. If they love their bodies, they move them. A sense of well-being comes from kinesthetic sensations, such as lifting, gliding and floating; from taking risks and discovering new capacities; from releasing anger, practicing self-discipline, or overcoming frustration. When mind and body are united through exercise, a person can experience a unique feeling of fulfillment as a total being. (1)

Unhealthy uses of exercise are focusing mainly on weight loss. Shaping up primarily to shape down can be disappointing. Whether exercise will reduce weight depends on the kind and duration of activity. In reality, building muscle does not

19

guarantee a smaller or lighter body. Those who are preoccupied with the scale miss many of the other positive benefits that movement offers. Another unhealthy use is focusing on competition. If a person finds themselves constantly competing with themselves or others in their exercise regime, they are defeating the purpose. It's an activity that's merely an extension of a highly competitive lifestyle that only adds another stress to the day. Movement that's strictly goal-oriented can be oppressive — and even dangerous — when exercisers push themselves beyond natural limitations. (2)

Exercise in and of itself should be enough to satisfy anyone who is truly in it to benefit themselves. Exercise is a way to connect to the inner self and realize the potential existing within. It is a way to break self-inflicted mental barriers and overcome personal obstacles to become the person that is the dream, that is the fantasy.

Exercise brings to life the vision that everything is possible through hope and belief and hard work. Consistency, time and commitment pay off to rewards that many do not believe. It is hard for many to take that mental leap and bring forth into reality a dream that is not so impossible.

To be fit, to be well, to be whole. It is what you can become through exercise. The mind is freed from the day-to-day hassles of feebleness, obesity, fatigue, worry and stress. It can soar to levels undocumented and take leave from a society bogged down in counting calories and measuring portions. Exercise transcends that realm of gym classes and just becomes another way to grow and test the limits that are placed on the human soul only by human society.

The Hippocrates Institute has seminars, teachers, instructors and others who can help a person take that leap of faith, to believe in the power of their bodies so they can believe in the power of their minds. But first, they must picture themselves where they want to be, because only through seeing where they want to be can they ultimately arrive there.

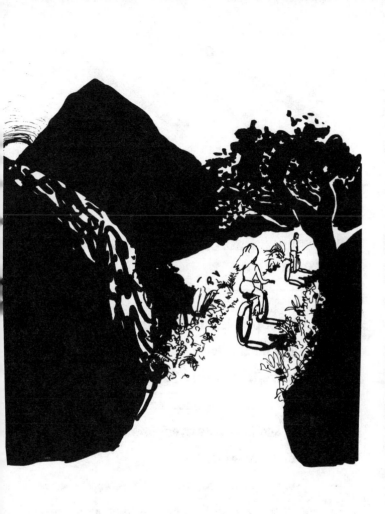

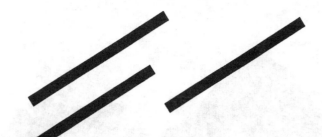

CHAPTER 4

Resistance Exercise: Why it is Necessary

Most people put in a videotape at 7 a.m. and bounce up and down. But that is only aerobic exercise. While it is very important and will be addressed later, resistance exercise is just as important and is grossly overlooked by a majority of the "civilized world."

It is estimated, in North America and Europe, that less than 5 percent of the populations are doing any kind of resistance exercise on a regular basis which will build their bodies. What many people do not understand is that resistance exercise is not confined to the thick-necked, muscle-clogged bodybuilders they see on television posing in competitions. Regular people who are not bulked up or tossing down high-protein drinks also need their fair share of resistance training, which can come in many acceptable, extremely doable forms.

Although many people have turned to expensive weight-training systems or free-weight workouts to build strength and muscle bulk, gymnasts, who use only their own bodies, prove conclusively that using one's own body weight as the resistance can result in very strong and beautifully proportioned bodies. Another thing about using one's own body as resistance is that very little apparatus is required. (3) In other words, expenses at a gym or investing in home equipment or other devices is not necessary. The human body will serve itself well, along with a little gravity and a few pieces of equipment.

Each of the following exercises should be done in continuous rhythm and reach a comfortable fatigue level to be effective. Pain, no matter what some fanatic exercise instructors say, is not a benefit to exercise, nor is it an immediate by-product. In fact, like in all other circumstances of life, pain should be avoided whenever possible. The exercises, which are familiar to almost everyone, are push-ups, pull-ups, abdominal exercises, back extension, the rowing machine, the military press, jump rope and bar dips. (4) The push-ups work the chest and shoulders; the rowing concentrates on the back and lower back. Abdominal exercises, like crunches, slim the waist; and the back extension elongates and strengthens the torso. The military press and bar dips also work the chest and arms, while the jump rope strengthens the legs, ankles and feet.

All of the movements are simple and easy. But more than that, they are effective. They build the muscle in the torso, legs, arms and back by using gravity and functional movements. It may be fun to work out with shiny, high-tech machines, but using a person's own body weight and these resistance exercises will develop strength in all major muscle groups of the body and will result in a well-proportioned physique. (5) In most cases, these exercises work faster and more effectively than any other exercise created by man.

If a person chooses to use weights, such as barbells or resistant training equipment, they have a long history of people before them who did the same thing. The origin of weight lifting was born in Venice, California many years ago by people realizing that when they picked up heavy weights, the body started to build their muscular structure.

Each person must decide for themselves which strategy best fits their lifestyle. The only thing each person must keep in mind is the benefit derived from resistance training. The advantage is both psychological and physiological, that is, resistance exercise helps develop the mind and the body.

First, consider the scenario of one person who has not exercised in a while. Then consider again, that most people can do a lot more than they think. It is simply a matter of approaching it with what the Hippocrates Institute asks everyone to approach life and healing — with an open mind.

If you were asked to lift your body up, by pulling with your arms, could you? In most cases, yes. That is psychology. Most people can imagine that they will accomplish something so simple, and through the same belief a person can imagine lifting their own body weight. So, in time this will happen. After one week, a person can most likely do one lift. After two weeks, they should be able to do two. Three weeks, etc., etc. Ultimately, a time comes when that person who could only do one lift is completing exercises of eight repetitions, three or four times, which starts to build muscle at a greater rate.

This type of exercise is ideal because it can be accomplished almost anywhere at anytime. For an extremely small investment, a bar can be bought for the exercises mentioned earlier. Anyone can do these exercises. It does not require massive amounts of skill or coordination or fitness. People who are recovering from accidents, who do not even have full use of their arms and legs, can do some of these exercises. Everyone is capable at any age.

The theory is that if one is comfortable with exercise, then they are able to do it. If something looks burdensome or more than one is capable of doing, then that person is more apt not to do it. Every single person is capable of doing one exercise once, be it a sit-up, push-up, stomach crunch or dip. So what that one person needs to learn is to start and know they can accomplish that one exercise, repeat it, until they become strong and achieve strength and self-confidence. Once a person starts to achieve these things, they start to build self-esteem, and then they want (and are able) to do more and more and more. It's a rolling ball. And as the saying goes, a rolling ball gathers no moss.

Repetition and consistency are also important when starting and achieving exercise. Not many people know that when a person who is incapable of performing an exercise pushes themselves to do one repetition that that rep is equal to another fit person doing three hours of exercise. For example, if a person who was in sedentary shape was paired with an exercise physiologist in great shape and they both exercised, the sedentary person's one repetition would benefit them as much as the physiologist's routine of three hours.

This is the basis of common sense and a higher power. Nothing is out of one's reach if you simply put forth an effort and believe. It is all a matter of belief. When a person who watches television and sits the majority of the day begins to exercise, the benefits are immediate. There are few things in life that bring immediate gratification — exercise is one of them. The muscles start tingling and aching. Tendons begin to stretch and give. Bones start to strengthen. The mind becomes filled with all the possibilities this motion can bring. In weeks or even days, the transformation from couch potato to living human being takes place. The energy begins to activate and push out the toxins and harmful residues that have taken up residence in the body. The heart begins to pump and the lungs fill with air. Sometimes, this process can come as a jolt to a system that has lain dormant for so long.

Imagine starting a car that sat idle for years. It is a dusty, rusty relic. But can it run? With a little care, maintenance, fuel and energy, of course it can. The human body is the same way, but most people treat their cars better than they treat their bodies. Give it fuel, give it energy. Then turn the key and watch it go!

Now, back to resistance exercise. What is the basic purpose besides building muscle mass? Not much. Because muscle mass is so extremely important, resistance exercise only needs that solitary purpose. Muscle mass helps the body battle the ravages of time: the one clock people cannot turn back, that bends the body and wilts the structure, if the bones and ligaments are not kept firm and limber. In one study of women over 65 years old, two groups were studied: The group of women who had exercised all their lives and the group who had not. In the group of senior women who had exercised since they were teenagers, only 7 percent of these women had osteoporosis, a degenerative disease that weakens the bones, causing them to bend. This statistic is versus the 90 percent of women who had not exercised, who also had the disease.

Resistance exercise also benefits the ligaments, the stretchy fibers of the body that connect the muscles and the organs. If the body is without muscular coordination and mass, then the organs that are held in place by the ligaments are left without support. Without support, the organs which bodies depend upon for functioning, are not operating correctly.

These are the very simple and down-to-earth reasons why resistance exercises are so important: not to impress the ladies or attract the men, but to insure a healthy, operational body that will weather the test of time and lengthen its keeper's time here. But even with these good reasons staring them in their faces, people can still manufacture reasons not to exercise. The list is long and generous: "I don't know if I can do that." "I have a bad back." "I live in a cold climate." "I don't have fins that are going to resist properly in the water." Those rank in credibility with "My hair hurts" and "My teeth itch." As it was mentioned before, those with physical challenges exercise. They lift weights. They work out. They do dips. They do stomach crunches.

They do all this because they are supposed to and because they can. Now people who are confined to wheelchairs, seriously impaired, have artificial limbs or learning disabilities, they, more than anyone else, should come up with excuses of why they cannot exercise. Anything they come up with will sound more valid than any excuse coming from the mouth of one who is simply lazy and uninformed. But do the physically challenged excuse themselves from life? Most do not. Most do not view themselves as less than capable because their body is less than 100 percent.

It is not within the physical body that the transformation should take place. Everyone has a mind. That is where the first challenge of exercise must be fought and won: No more "I can't" or "I won't." Life should be a constant series of "I can" and "I will." Otherwise, where is the conquest of negativity? Where is the gain and joy of living life to the fullest? Where is the triumph? Ask the physically challenged. The man on crutches or the woman without hands, and they'll answer. It is with the correct attitude that any problem can be solved. And the biggest difficulty is usually within the soul, within the mind and within the spirit.

Once that is overcome, anything is possible.

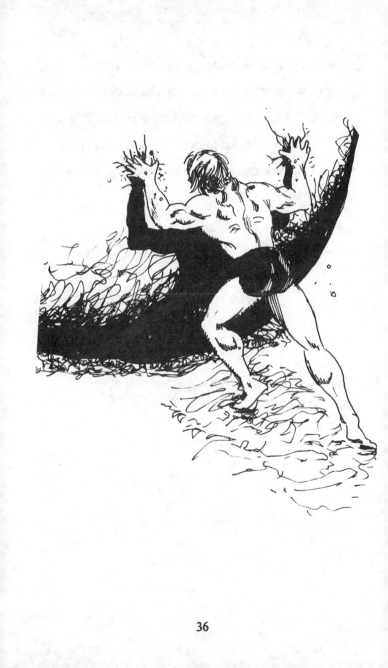

CHAPTER 5

Aerobic Exercise: It is More Than Just Bouncing Up and Down

Once upon a time, when people thought of aerobics, they thought of jogging. Running at a low intensity is not for everyone, nor should it be. Jogging is only one form of aerobics; there are many more. But first, what are aerobics and why are they so important?

We've discussed the importance of resistance exercise: muscular tone, organ function, self-esteem and strength.

Aerobic exercise has the same benefits. Aerobic exercise means steady exercise, exercise that demands an uninterrupted output from the muscles for a particular amount of time. It has been shown in many exercise-physiology laboratories that steady, continuous exercise repeated every day reverses the syndrome of fat replacing muscle more quickly than any other type of exercise. (6)

The word aerobic means air, specifically the oxygen in the air. The muscles need oxygen to function, and their need for oxygen goes up dramatically when they are worked. (7) So aerobics in a nutshell are continuous exercises that require more than the normal amount of air. An extra large intake of oxygen benefits the circulatory and respiratory system, enlivens the blood and the brain, literally by sending more oxygen in that direction and releasing the toxins and poisons in the system through exhaling, sweating and relieving other waters from the system. Is it any wonder why our bodies crave water while we exercise? It wants to replace the dirty with the clean. With clean water flowing in, the contaminated waters flow out, leaving the body tiredly refreshed and cleansed.

But aerobics are not confined to fad videotapes, crowded gym classes or the beloved jogging. More than any other form of exercise, aerobics ushers in a wealth of fun, which can be fascinating and creative.

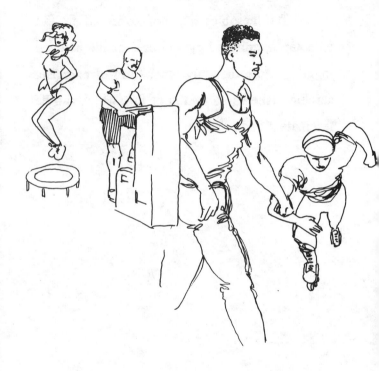

CHAPTER 6

Choices, Choices, Choices: The Many Forms of Aerobic Exercise

---

Running

The most obvious choice is running. With the exception of vigorous swimming or cross-country skiing, running can be one of the best cardiovascular exercises available. Unlike cycling or swimming, which are antigravity sports that use the water or the bike to support the entire body, running forces the person to use their major muscle groups just to keep upright. Because these muscles in large part determine the aerobic workload, running has an immediate and undeniable advantage in making a workout aerobic. Running is also independent and convenient. It doesn't take a group to go running, only a good location and sturdy pair of shoes. When one is running, he or she must remember to find a grassy or earthy surface to exercise on to prevent the jolting of bones and joints from running on hard pavement.

Finally, running is the least expensive sport to participate in. Even though good running shoes are fairly expensive, the financial outlay is still considerably less than a health club membership, a year of aerobics classes or resort skiing, and is one of the best ways to improve a person's aerobic base. (8)

Swimming

If a person doesn't know how to swim, he or she should learn. It is the safest of all exercises.

No jarring motions, no hard surfaces and hopefully in an ozone-clear, pristine pool. All one needs is a pair of goggles so they can open their eyes under water without suffering the sting of chlorine or salt, a tight-fitting nylon swimsuit that will reduce the drag in the water, and if necessary a bathing cap and they're off.

Swimming is also the closest thing to a natural challenge we humans have. The resistance of the water forces our lungs to expand, our heart to pump and our muscles to push. Swimming in a body of water is also in flow with the natural rhythm of body development. When a swimmer wants to rest, they do not stretch by the side of the road or place their bike under the shade of a tree. They simply turn onto their backs and float, much like they did in their mother's belly before they were born. A pool is also a place for fun and good times. A little splash and a little spray and it's all about laughter and joviality.

Bicycling

Next is bicycling. Bicycling, as mentioned before, is an antigravity sport which can be preferable to running, aerobic dancing or tennis for some because of the jarring and eccentric stresses these exercises can place on the musculoskeletal system, which can lead to soreness and sometimes injuries. But in cycling, the bike supports the weight. As a result, the jarring forces associated with the weight-bearing sports are drastically reduced.

Cycling also requires the use of huge muscle masses and thus is an excellent aerobic sport. It involves all the muscles of the legs and muscles of the hips and lower trunk. Even though the arms and shoulders are not used as much as they are in running, for example, it is still an extremely effective way to achieve cardiovascular fitness. (9)

Skiing

If a person is living in the kind of climate that provides snow every winter and lots of it, then they can add skiing to their list of aerobic possibilities. Cross-country skiing is much more exciting and accessible with the advent of manicured trails, improved gear and upgraded sportswear. With the creation of roller skis, snow isn't even a must.

Cross-country skiing is an affordable sport, usually costing one-third to one-half less than downhill skiing. Equally important, it is a very safe sport. The flexibility of the foot in the ski lessens the likelihood of an ankle or knee sprain. It is a great sport for those who claim it is just too cold out to exercise. (10)

Walking

And of course, there's walking. Anyone can do this exercise. We've been doing it since we were 1 year old. One foot in front of the other and that's it. Like running, the most it takes is the outdoors, or a treadmill, and a good pair of shoes to be fully equipped and ready. The essence of walking, however, is thinking. Being outdoors in a new surrounding, breathing in the air and taking in the scenery, and allowing the mind to simply do what it does best: wander and contemplate.

All these exercises allow a person to do that. Imagine biking cross-country, where only the trees line the path; or skiing over a snow-clogged wilderness, taking in the frigid winds, feeling the sun bounce off the ice and onto your skin; or swimming in the ocean, off a beach. All these exercises are more than just independent ventures to build a better body; they are an opportunity to explore and to connect.

Women walking together, laughing and chatting about the day's events. Letting off some steam and working their muscles at the same time. When a family goes to the pool to swim, rarely do they swin continuously. They talk, interact, listen and play. And when a man goes running, early in the morning, just as others are stretching themselves awake, what does he do? Meditate to the steady slap of his sneakers against the pavement, planning his day, clearing his mind, concentrating on his glide and building his heart.

Outdoor exercise has a domino effect in a life. Not only does it improve the body, it serves the soul a daily dose of air and light. It gives the mom a chance to look beyond the day's chores and introduce her baby in the stroller to the wonderful world of peace and tranquillity mixed with energy and action. Exercise should also be about expanding horizons.

Strapping on a pair of rollerblades for the first time gives the hard and fast gym dweller a taste of adventure. Daring the conventional runner to test his skills on a trampoline is daring him to test his self-confidence and inner strength. What will the average exerciser do when introduced to the concept of rebounding: a form of exercise that requires bouncing on a mini-trampoline to cleanse the lymphatic system, fortify the circulatory system and empower the respiratory system? If they are truly interested in benefiting from exercise, they will embrace new concepts, such as rebounding. By asking the questions: Can I do this? Will I succeed? They succeeded, and they credit a daily dose of rebounding, eating well and positive thinking to their recovery from injuries and obesity.

Exercise is a thinking person's game. It never stops. The challenge to overcome doubts, worries, anxieties and fear is the basis of exercise. And when that person who runs, cycles, rebounds, swims, walks, rollerblades or dances looks at themselves and what they've accomplished, they can only ask one thing of themselves: more.

If the outdoors are not available, say it's raining, sleeting, hailing, or there is a hurricane watch in effect, no one expects an exerciser to reap the benefits of the outdoors then. Many indoor aerobic exercises make it possible for a person to get a good workout and cleanse their body without leaving their home or gym.

In almost all gyms, stair climbing machines and bench stepping classes are the rage. Although the machines won't make a person any more fit than actually using the stairs, they do offer some plusses, such as continuous uphill work and freedom from the concern of exercising in a deserted, potentially dangerous stairwell. Jumping rope is also a simple option that most people have forgotten that they know how to do.

If a person runs as their form of aerobic exercise, then jumping rope is a great substitute for when that person travels to an unknown place and would prefer not to run in unknown neighborhoods. An employee could take their 15-minute coffee break by jumping rope, or a traveler could jump rope quietly in his hotel room. Although jumping rope is a bit too strenuous on the joints to be used every day, it is a good replacement when conditions are such that staying indoors is the best choice.

Walking doesn't always require an outdoors either. Since the invention of the treadmill, a large population of people are now setting the controls and taking a long, brisk walk indoors, while listening to music, reading a book or watching the evening news. The best pace on a treadmill is a fast walk or a slow jog.

Rebounding, discussed earlier, uses the mini-trampoline to aerobicize the heart. A person can vary their workout on the trampoline by running in place on it, jumping rope or dancing to music on it.

Music can add a whole new dimension to any exercise; sometimes music can become the exercise, as is the case with aerobic dancing. Now, when people think of aerobics, they usually think of a room full of people in workout clothes bouncing to some technophonic hit. But these days, aerobic dancing is that and a lot more. There is step aerobics, which uses a bench that is adjustable in height to resist gravity and create more of a pull on the lower body. The classes not only teach fitness, they teach coordination, rhythm, concentration and motion. Low impact aerobics, in which the feet never leave the ground, and high impact, which involves a lot of jumping and bouncing, can be custom tailored to fit the needs of the individual.

Because aerobic dancing uses both upper and lower body muscles, a person will burn as much or more fat as they would running. The classes use a variety of foot movements, so there is a reduction in the risk of repetition-induced trauma. And because they're just plain fun, the "sticking to it" potential is far greater than with most other aerobic sports. (11) Plus, there is a room full of people participating, making socialization and enjoyment much higher.

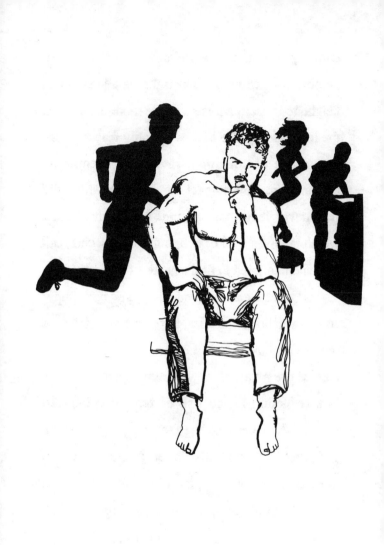

CHAPTER 7

How to Start Exercising

The rules of exercising are to have fun, have fun and have more fun. But to have fun, a person must first begin. Otherwise, they'll never know what they're missing.

Once a person starts they should remember a few helpful hints that will keep them in the game and bring them back for more:

1.   If you cannot do it right, do it often. People sometimes get too hung up on rules. They

overlook the fact that a whole lot of "not quite aerobic" exercise can be just as good as a moderate amount of true aerobic exercise. If you can't exercise exactly by the rules or exactly in the correct form, who cares? Just continue to exercise and do not use the lack of perfect as an excuse to quit. Exercise a lot. Quantity can substitute for quality. That's why those who play sports are often in better shape than those who strictly exercise at a health club.

2. Do not exercise with a fit friend. If a person is just starting out, is really overweight or out of shape, it will be too hard on their body to try to maintain the same routine as a fit friend. Also with the best of intentions, fit friends push the not-so-fit friend too fast, too often or too hard because it's so easy for them. The sedentary person ends

up getting injured and possibly stopping, while they think the exercise was worthless. Start slow and build slow. In the end the body that has been created is a masterpiece of time, effort and commitment, not a get-fit-quick regime.

3. Start slowly. It needs to be emphasized that gentle exercise pays off. If you are exercising at a slow pace, one that is 65 percent of your maximum heart rate, your body will adapt and profit from the exercise. You may just be walking and it may not seem like much to you or your friends, but at night as you sleep, your body will say, "She doesn't exercise very hard, but she sure does a lot of it. I'd better adapt to this." And adapt successfully it will.

4. Exercise as often as possible. Lots of books claim that we need to exercise for a half hour at a time. In the end, the rule should be to get out there and exercise as

much as you possibly can. If you really want to know what to do, find a 12-year-old boy and do whatever he does. When he rolls on the floor, you roll on the floor. If he goes for a bike ride, you go for a bike ride. If you keep up at his pace, it won't be long before you're pretty darn fit. Get the idea? Do a lot.

5.   Do not even think about distance. If you're thinking about this, you're missing the point of exercise. It doesn't matter how far you run, walk, swim or cycle. What matters is how many minutes a day you spend trying to change your body into a fit body. Exercise for time, not distance. When you exercise for time, you have two advantages. First, you don't need a measured course or track. All you need is a watch. Second, you aren't tempted to exercise too hard. Somebody once remarked that we ought to match exercise minutes with the number

of minutes we eat. Just think how many minutes a day you spend eating. If you were to match even half those minutes doing exercise, you would be fitter than a fox. Ask yourself, "Am I putting in enough time each day to expect my body to change in a positive way?" If the answer is not what you'd like, then incorporate exercise into your lifestyle as a given, not as a scheduled item that is optional depending upon the weather, the television or your mood.

6. Cold weather is not an excuse. Cross-country skiing, playing in the snow, building a snowman, sledding, snowball fights, walks in a winter wonderland. All those things we do in the cold without harm, simply because they're fun. Why should exercise be any different?

7. Rain is not an excuse either. Running in the

rain is fun. Go out and get wet and come back and jump in the shower. It's a wonderful experience. Some of you do not want to exercise in bad weather because you're afraid you'll fall on the slippery roads, or you'll catch a cold or your hair will be ruined. Fine. Put an aerobics exercise tape in the VCR, or get on your stationary bike or go to the gym. No excuses.

8.   Find a sport or make one. People who make a sport out of their exercise have a real advantage. For example, if you compare 100 people who use outdoor bicycles with 100 who use stationary bikes, you will find that the outdoor bicycle people are much more fit, and usually are a lot happier. Why is this? There are many reasons, but the most obvious one is that nobody gets on an outdoor bike for only 15 minutes. Once you get on a bike, the

inclination is to go much farther than you can go in that time. You just keep going and going because it's half exercise and half fun. Another reason outdoor bicyclists are more fit is that outdoor bicycling is associated with friends. You do lots of outings not because you need the exercise but because you like to do things with your friends.

9. Do not diet. Most people think of dieting as deprivation. It seems that in America all we think about is eating fewer calories and going on "diets." If you eat well, filling your body with organic, wholesome foods from the Earth, then calorie-counting, portion-measuring, fat-pinching and diet-fadding will become obsolete.

10. Eat often. Out-of-shape people who go without food experience drops in blood sugar over and over during the day, and these drops precipitate hunger or

depression. If you are out of shape, you have a special need to keep that blood sugar up by eating often. You shouldn't resort to gimicky diets or skipping meals or fasting. You should eat foods that are low in fat, high in complex carbohydrates and packed with energy. Meatless, greaseless diets serve the body best, cleansing it with organic fibers and rejuvenating it with oxygen and power. So despite the latest diet book, eating well can benefit the body. Just eat the right things.

11.   If you have any more questions, ask a fox. Translated, that means get out and go. For example, don't worry about the time of day for exercise. Do you ask a fox what time of day he does his aerobic exercise? Do you ask a 12-year-old girl when she bikes or runs? Do you tell your dog to be sure to do his aerobics at 10 a.m. every day? The point is, fit creatures exercise a lot. They

get out and go. They don't worry about the time of day. If you are a morning person, exercise in the morning. If you are an evening person, exercise in the evening. Do not let someone with a Ph.D. tell you that a certain time of day is better than any other time of day. The right time is up to you and your personality.

12.   People who skip a day's exercise are not useless, lazy or hopeless. So that removes just about everyone from the pile. We all get lazy and skip a day. In fact, lots of us take a week off now and then. If you do not exercise for a day, do not feel bad about it. Just get back to it when you can, knowing that everyone is like that. Everyone has a busy life that calls for a tendency toward children or careers or study or simply relaxing. Exercise is a part of life that will forever remain important and not forgotten simply because one workout was skipped

or one walk was left untread. Do not be too rigid about the rules — remember, exercise is fun! (12)

Also when a person starts exercising, they should keep two more things in mind. Ask friends to join and make up a sport if the ones that are around do not fit your criteria. Exercise is a full process that takes in all that the world has to offer: love, friendship, warmth and generosity. Sharing the gift of fitness, well spirits and good times is such a wonderful present that exercise, unless it is a time for reflection and meditation, should be shared with friends and family.

People are great motivators. Two can chat about the world's events or the latest headlines while walking around the neighborhood. Mother and daughter can join an aerobics class together. Son and father can play a vigorous game of catch or tennis. Exercise is a time to share and enjoy and experience life with love and warmth. What better time to interact than during a sporting match when wits are sharp and alertness is high, when you're in tune with the energy and the spirit flowing through you. The strength and the power is there, so take advantage of it and use it to connect with those that are loved and cherished.

Lastly, when beginning an exercise program, do not be discouraged if the perfect exercise for you does not exist. The treadmill was an invention, as was the rollerblade, mini-trampoline and bicycle. Who's to say that from your mind won't emerge another great idea that will lift exercise to another realm? Not everyone is a runner, nor is everyone a swimmer, a walker, a dancer or a biker. If people are not happy with these choices, they should survey the land and take inventory of what they want versus what is available, then create the perfect vehicle that will enable them to exercise to the fullest enjoyment possible. Exercise in and of itself is about pushing boundaries and transforming the conventional. It is about expanding the mind and increasing life's possibilities. So if the machine that you want does not exist, create it. If the shoe to make running a joy is not being sold, invent it. And use the mind to increase the level of exercise.

If a person believes they can, they will. Exercise is simply a process that demonstrates this phenomenon over and over and over again.

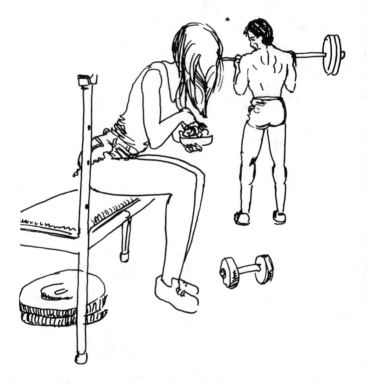

CHAPTER 8

Primitive Cultures — Fit Lifestyles

This society does not approach exercise properly. We write books. We talk on talk shows and we listen to every doctor who says this is what we are supposed to be doing, instead of doing what comes naturally, instead of listening to instinct, instead of listening to nature.

In most undeveloped parts of the world, people do not have gyms or treadmills or exercise gurus telling them how beneficial a morning walk is. People exercise daily because it is in rhythm with everything that is natural and whole.

In a small region of the Andes mountains, all the people lived to be over 100 years old, and they primarily eat living, oxygenated food. This is part of the reason they stay alive so long and remain so vibrant and healthy. People in their 90s run up cliffs in this region, scaling mountains with a 10-degree angle and not breaking a sweat. They run all day long, using their limbs and heart to run 20 miles over valleys, mountains and hills. And they smile the entire time. No wrinkles on their faces. No cancer or chronic immune deficiency. Very little sickness.

The reason is because their lifestyles are unpolluted, unhibited, unrestrained and stress free, which allows them to do what comes instinctively. Exercise is embedded in a human's soul right next to love, peace and creation. Exercise is a part of ourselves that we are taught to ignore not long after grade school. Interests turn to money-making, relationship-building, family, career, washing the car, calling your mother, shopping for groceries and paying the bills. A host of excuses not to exercise is created as it is relegated to a sub-important position. Primitive cultures do not worry about missing the next television special and therefore put off going to the gym. They do not even have gyms, where hundreds of people gather in an air-conditioned place and get on machines to do what's natural.

Cultures not overcome by modern development have not forgotten what is essential and important, so they exercise freely and generously, living long and living well. In exercise, they develop a huge sense of self-confidence and self-esteem that our culture tries to buy in self-help books. Things that benefit the body must come from nature, not some publishing company. Look within to find the answer to begin the journey to wellness and well-being.

With that kind of benchmark, anything can be accomplished. For example, this society has athletes who train strenuously for years, decades even, to compete in the Olympic Games. They are the best urban society has to offer in the way of athletic prowess and agility and strength. But put these modern-trained athletes up against any person from a primitive culture, which probably doesn't even know that the Olympics exist, and, hands down, the primitive person would beat the Olympian. Why?

Because they are endowed with a belief that all that goes into making an Olymic winner just comes naturally. So from birth, instead of training for a dream to compete, they trained for life. It wasn't a matter of the fastest time or the longest yard. It was a matter of having fun, being fit to enjoy life and sharing that enjoyment with others. We have overlooked these cultures because we perceive them as unknowledgable.

They are not sophisicated. They do not drive or attend operas or go to sporting events. And because of our perception we are missing out on a reality that could be helpful in finding the key to such tranquility and peace.

Sometimes we need not look farther than our own back door to find what is hidden in the lost recesses of the world. Primitive cultures laugh and play and smile when they exercise. It is a game. It is recreation and sport. Everyone knows of at least one person who takes this same approach to exercise: a child. If you want to see it in action, follow an eight-year-old child around for a couple of days. There's no such thing as a quiet child. At the dinner table, they rock their chairs. They fuss and fidget when you try to teach them a game of cards. To them, walking is ridiculous — it's easier to run. If we adults skipped and pranced the way kids do all the time, we wouldn't need to read all these books on how to become fit. Children do not consciously seek out extra exercise. They just do it because it's the easiest, fastest and most convenient way to do things. To them, it's more fun to be moving than to be still. (13)

And that's how all adults should approach exercise: as a childhood experience re-lived. It is a form of liberation and freedom: of times when stress and overachieving weren't the main goals of the day. Exercise takes us back to when skipping ropes and playing leapfrog were just fun, not exercise; to when our mothers told us to go outside and play. And six hours later, when the sun was setting and the mosquitos were biting, we come back in full of life, covered with sweat and glowing with energy.

That's how exercise is supposed to feel — energized, like every muscle is responding to a wake-up call and the brain is moving to a rhythm filled with oxygen and coursing blood. Exercise is a mode of transporation. It takes us back to childhood and forward into expansion.

It enlivens our bodies as well as our souls and lifts the burden of daily existence if just for a little while. Sorting out a problem is easier when all you have to think about is the next step of a walk or the next lap in a pool. Counting the reps in a resistance workout clears the mind of distracting material and instead concentrates on making all the joints and muscles and bones work in coordination to lift that next weight or do that next crunch. All that is in the mind is fitness and how to become better. How to reach that next goal and better oneself just a little more.

Exercise is the celebration of love, prosperity and freedom. As mentioned in previous chapters, it is a basic natural tenet of life, practiced long before it was discussed and analyzed. It builds the heart and cleans the body. It can be done alone as a form of meditation and reflection or as part of a family interaction. It takes the exerciser back to the days of endless energy, yet propels them forward with challenges that their body will meet someday.

Exercise is more than simply moving the body. It is moving the mind and moving the life to a better, higher place.

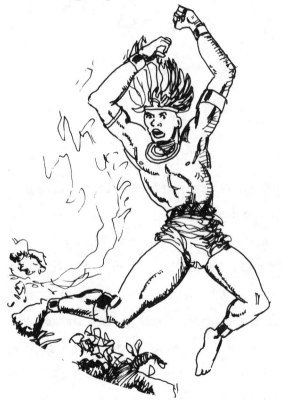

CHAPTER 9

The Abuses of Exercise

Can we overdo exercise? Yes, we can. And more often than not, we do. Exercise for some is a way to deal with life. And exercise should be only a part of life. It is not a cure-all, and it can be abused and misused like so many other things in today's society. Exercise can do a lot of things. Not only the spiritual, mental and emotional advantages mentioned previously, but physically as well. It can help control weight, reduce depression and anxiety, increase self-esteem, lower the risk of cardiovascular disease, ease lower back pain and promote strength, endurance and flexibility. But when abused, exercise has the potential to injure, promote pain and fatigue, cause heart problems, compound emotional problems and disappoint the exerciser. (14)

Always keep in mind why you are exercising: to fulfill a part of your life that is natural, to expand horizons and broaden perspectives. Exercise does not cure problems, but it does offer a forum in which to sort out problems. Exercise does not make us the person in the commercial or on the magazine cover, but it does help us become the best we can be, which should always be enough. Exercise is not a permanent solution to serious mental situations, such as depression, but it can offer a temporary stay from the depression through the natural lift of endorphins. Exercise is not a magical potion that can be taken and that will wipe away all the ills. It is part of a regime of healthy living, positive attitude, wholesome eating, mental exercise and general well-being. It is one part of many that make a whole, happy life and should not be abused, overused or ruined trying to make it more than what it is.

Justly, exercise can be used as a positive alternative to many other addictive behaviors because it is incompatible with negative activities, such as overeating, smoking and drinking. Exercise is very often a component of addiction treatment programs because it can aid in the process of recovering from negative activities and it provides an excellent way to recover self-esteem and to develop a sense of mastery over one's self and one's environment. (15)

Exercise can be used as an avoidance manuever for those people who do not want to deal with other aspects of their lives. While exercise does enable a person to grow and expand through challenge, meditation and accomplishment, other facets of living — work, love and relaxation —

also help a person grow and should not be substituted with exercise. As stated before, exercise is just one important part of a whole, balanced and spiritually complete life.

Instead of dealing with life on its terms and taking control with a can-do attitude, some people may hide behind the cloak of exercise, postponing or avoiding other activities, such as relationships or career advancement, because they are too afraid. Just as the alcoholic hides in liquor or the drug addict retreats behind a high, so too do exercise abusers schedule their lives around exercise, hoping the problems will take care of themselves or simply go away.

Life is full of experiences we would all like to avoid if we could. Some people avoid establishing or maintaining personal relationships, intimacy and social contact, while others try to dodge marital, parental, financial or career responsibilities. After a period of encounters with disagreeable experiences, it's completely natural to want to stop the unpleasantness. (16) But hiding out from life on the treadmill or making excuses by saying you have to go running is not the way.

Exercise should be used as a tool to help a person overcome their shortcomings and help them realize that they can cope with anything that life deals them, not as an escape mechanism. The whole pyschology behind exercise is to overcome the first hurdle so you can conquer the second. When people do not understand the principles behind exercise, its pyschology and universal connection, they abuse it. To stop retreating into the world of exercise, slowly face the problems and deal with them one at a time, until the whole thing doesn't look so big. But don't hide from the world. It can be controlled and managed with the correct outlook, patience and understanding.

Another abuse that people take out on exercise is taking all the fun out of it. Rigid schedules and carefully maintained rituals take the spontaneity out of running around the block in the rain or going swimming when friends come to visit unannounced. People who strive for perfection, setting every little milestone of a workout into granite, also miss its purpose. They are using a natural function to ignore feelings of anxiety and dissatisfaction instead of using that natural function to think of a natural solution to beat these feelings.

Exercise should not be a scheduled, fixed event. It should be as common as blinking and as instinctual as putting our hands out to catch ourselves when we fall. Looking at exercise from a narrow view also narrows the view of life and what it can offer. If you never venture outside the realm of what is established, how can you ever know what else exists?

Test the boundaries, push the limit. Try new things at different times. If a person always walked in the morning, they would never see the sunset. If a person always jogged in the afternoon, they would never feel the mist of new morn dew. If a person only went to the gym 90 minutes every day and did the treadmill, weights and stretching, how would they learn the benefits of floating in a pool, rollerblading in the park or playing volleyball on the beach?

Exercise comes in as many different forms and combinations as people. So why abuse it by limiting it?

The final abuse of exercise is using it to try to become something that we're not. Exercise will not give a short person long legs. It will not give a blond person brown hair and it will not remove the effects of genetics, which dictates who is short, tall, slight or big-boned. Mom, Dad and their family lines supply the material and God chooses where it will appear and on whom. All exercise which we do is physically improving the current package. And if self-love is already there, then an improvement upon a good situation is nothing but better.

A psychologically healthy view of exercise is one that says, "I'm exercising to stay in shape, but I know that my body size, whether heavy or thin, doesn't dictate who I am or what kind of person I am." However, if a person is abusing exercise, their view would probably be "If only my abdomen were flat, people would like me. If only my thighs were slimmer, I'd like myself. If only my body were smaller, I'd be happy." For those whose abuse is rooted in poor body image, the exercise program does not stem only from a physical need to drop some weight, it grows from pathological attempts at self-improvement. (16)

But self-improvement, just like exercise, does not start with what one sees in the mirror. Self-improvement begins inside with a sincere, wholehearted embrace of who you are and self-love that comes from who you were and can be; and this will add up to what you will become. Just like sychophants, kissing up to people for acceptance and warmth, abusers are looking to exercise to give them total self-love and self-worth. Now, exercise can improve and build self-esteem. Overcoming obstacles and constructing a firm, fit body is reason to be proud and confident, but these elements should not replace the inner workings of love and self-respect. Those have to be developed either separate from exercise and improved as a result of exercise. It's like building a house. Before you can improve the structure with paint and landscaping, there first must be a base of concrete, bricks, plumbing and wood. Without it, the improvements and expansion do not matter because there is nothing to improve or expand on.

Exercise helps a healthy person meet expectations and develop a sense of triumph and completion. But self-love must be instilled long before the first ball is thrown or the first weight is lifted.

Inner preparation must take place before true exercise can begin and become an essential ingredient in a whole life. Mentally, exercise requires an open playing field, uninhibited and spontaneous. Emotionally, exercise requires a love of self and a need to augment soul and spirit with a daily dose of liberation and youth. Psychologically, exercise requires the understanding of the challenge and how, when it is mastered, the self-esteem grows and confidence swells. And spiritually, exercise requires a belief in man's place in the universe and how that universe is filled with breathing, moving creatures that see exercise as a part of development and life. And that as an inhabitant of this universe, man must follow its rules and use his body in the way it was meant to be used. For love, for energy, for growth and for strength.

Abuse comes in many shapes and sizes. Some cannot believe that something so good for you can be abused, but our instincts regarding exercise have been grossly altered by messages and lessons taught by an ignorant society. We no longer know how to gauge when to stop, pushing ourselves for the wrong reasons to achieve a goal that will be there if we work hard or if we work leisurely to attain it.

Does it really matter how many months it took to run that mile as long as you had fun? Did this benefit you and did you grow as a result of the experience? Does it really matter that an ordinary woman who exercises as part of her life plan will never look like a supermodel? No. Does it really matter that a person is not competitive, not particularly good at any sport, has no coordination and cannot catch a ball? No, as long as his body receives the fruits of his fun. None of it matters a bit.

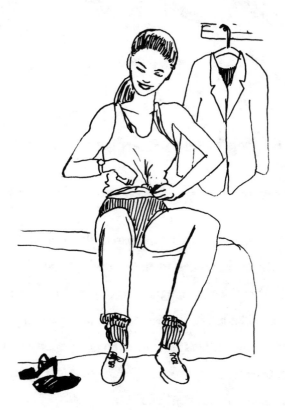

CHAPTER 10

Creating Time to Exercise

Exercise is a natural part of living. It makes us whole. It makes us feel good. It makes us complete. Such an integral part of your life should not be scheduled. If possible, make it your life's work. Teach others how to exercise properly and for the right reasons. Teach buoyancy and relaxation, fulfillment and esteem.

As unlikely as it may sound, some people do devote their lives to exercise. Not in the form of worship or religion, but just as a career choice, so that while completing a necessary function in life — exercising — they also can earn a living, make a difference and possibly change someone else's life: aerobic instructors, swimming teachers, golf pros, lifeguards, football players and gymnasium administrators. There are even those whose work indirectly gives them the benefit of exercise: the construction workers, gardeners, window washers and dog walkers. They all get their daily dose of exercise by going to work.

One man had spent a great majority of his life learning. He earned his Ph.D. and went on to become a professor. In the end, he hated it. Time spent grading exams and lecturing inside a building were not fulfilling his need to be physical, so he quit within two weeks of taking this professorship. His family was surprised to say the least because after that he went on to become a carpenter. Now he is happier than he ever was teaching, for two reasons that also apply to exercise. According to him, he starts a project and within a very short time he can stand back and see his accomplishments. The second thing is that he views his job as exercise he's being paid for. Some days, he said, clients pay him overtime and he feels guilty because all they did was allow him more time to exercise.

That is the kind of attitude that everyone should have. It should not be one where exercise is a chore that has to be eked out one hour every day. It is almost as if exercise has taken on the characteristics of religion. Most of today's society does not tolerate spirituality for more than one or two hours once a week: when we happen to check into our local church or temple, and we sit there and play that we are being spiritual. We dress in our best clothes, and we honor a higher power. We go through the motions without really grasping the purpose of our being there. While we are supposed to be praying, we're thinking about dinner, or the dry cleaning or what sport will be televised when we get home. We're not asking for anything, being grateful for anything or simply being humble.

Religion becomes a chore that is stuffed in between washing the car Saturday and getting dinner together Sunday.

Exercise has the same unpopular position. We have to expand beyond the trappings of 30 minutes a day, and make exercise something we do without a schedule. It has to become a part of life, like the foods we eat and books we read.

No matter what you're doing, make it an exercise. Dancing, going to pick up people at the airport, anything. Can you imagine the response if you suggested running from the gate to the car at the airport? It would invite serious inspection from those who expect a sedentary, customary stroll. But can you imagine the benefits of a spontaneous sprint? No one in the airport will mind. People run through airports all the time. And even if they do stare, they'll be staring at people who are youthful on the inside and could not care less if they look a little wacky. A child does not care when they dance or skip in the aisle of a plane. It's not about other people's perception of you. It's about your perception of yourself. And that perception will improve if exercise is made a vital component to the regular events of the day. If you get off a plane feeling drab and tired, run. If a movie went too long and left you feeling stiff and achy, stretch and jump in place. If work is wearing on the nerves, causing the shoulders to hunch around the ears, go for a brisk walk in the sunshine or the rain, around the building or around the block. It does not matter. Just move for motion's sake and get the blood pumping.

Or be a child. Think like a child, play with a child, laugh like a child and enjoy like a child. They have no worries, no cares if their life is secure and safe and happy. Of course, being an adult with adult responsibilities can make it difficult to shrug off the doldrums and relive infancy, but just for a moment try. The first thing that comes to mind as a child is exercise. Running, jumping, bouncing, playing. Dream of when school (or work) lets out and you can go home and play on the treadmill, in your aerobics class, in the weight room, in the pool. Children are often told to emulate us, the adults, when in fact it would be much more beneficial to the world as a whole if we emulated them.

Children grab each other's hands on the playground and swing them, exercising their arms and backs. Children hang upside down on the monkey bars, letting the blood rush to their brains, while they get a whole new perspective on the world. Children release tension by crying when they're hurt or laughing when they're happy, not holding emotions inside where they fester and sicken the body.

Children are examples from a higher power that give us insight to exercise, eating habits, learning abilities, spontaneity, and most of all, love. Children embrace the world with a hearty hug and announce their arrival with the strength of 10 bears. Adults should learn to throw themselves with such abandon into practices that help them grow and challenge them to succeed.

And adults would be lucky to be children.

Then again, adults can take advantage of their age and maturity by exercising in a way reserved strictly for those wise enough to do it well and reap the largest benefits: making love. Making love qualifies as the most engrossing, intense and passionate form of exercise known to man. It involves the mind, the soul and all parts of the body. It increases the heart rate, works the muscles and calls for ingenuity, creativity and skill: all things that a great athlete needs.

In the oriental philosophy, they talk about certain passionate exercises that are very subtle and that are shared between man and woman. These are called contra exerises, exercises that do not take a lot of movement, but do require 100 percent devotion from the mind and muscles. Making love totally sets a person free, much like the freedom of a child. It is a wondrous combination of intimacy, movement and exercise. Few people can ask more of an experience than complete involvement and complete fulfillment, and that is what making love provides. In addition to creating populations and expressing emotion, making love is a form of exercise that many people do not count in their daily regime to become fit. And that is a mistake that needs to be corrected. Making love is as natural and as much a part of this Earth as the food it produces.

When looking at food, for example, a perfect, well-balanced diet of food is supposed to be 100 percent symbiotically derived from the earth. A living diet is a combination of foods that are still alive when we eat them, so it produces energy once it enters the bloodstream, muscles and organs. In the same process of eating wherein the food is cooked, it is being depleted of its energy. The elements that make food beneficial literally go up in smoke — in the frying pan, in the oven, in the wok, in the microwave. Cooking food that is naturally alive, filled with nutrients and oxygen, interrupts the flow of nature from the earth into our bodies and the purpose of eating is missed.

The same holds true for exercise. Exercise should not interrupt the flow of the universe, and what is natural and good. Exercise should be a part of that flow.

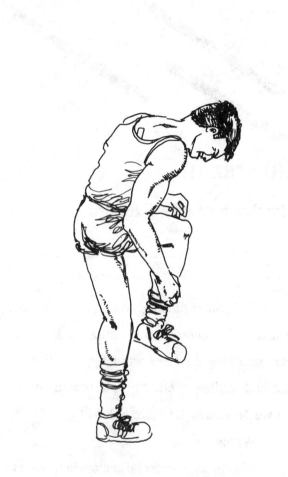

CHAPTER 11

The Psychology of Exercise

O.K., we're running. We know that is good because we're sweating, breathing hard, feeling alive, watching the trees whirl by, smelling the grass and smiling at other people running by us. And we only have 1.7 more miles to go.

Wrong.

We run until we feel like stopping. We run until we feel like walking or sprinting or jogging or talking with a friend. We do not restrict ourselves to a time, a place, a distance or a strict regime when we exercise because exercise is about freedom. And who can be free when they have 1.7 miles to go in 25 minutes, around the corner of Main and Elm, like they have run every day for the past two years? That is not freedom. That is boredom for the body and the brain. No challenge exists, no boundaries are movable. Instead of making exercise a time to expand, we changed it into another job, where a person shows up at 8 a.m. and leaves at 5 p.m., where he files the same papers, listens to the same complaints and eats at the same restaurant for lunch, every day, in and out, no change. No exploration, no risk, no gain.

If an exercise routine is varied, if new goals are set, the worst that can happen is that a new person emerges from you.

There is an abundance of truth in the statement that if people go through challenges, in spite of the possbility that they will fail, they will develop a sense of character that claims success as its destiny. In other words, in the process of trying and failing and trying again, a character is born and that character will reap success one day. Because with that kind of attitude and perseverance, life obstacles are overcome and left behind. It is just a matter of trying.

This outlook gives people the ability to prevail — a trait everyone could benefit from. Through trial and error, success and failure — trying and trying to swim two laps instead of one, running that much harder and faster and longer than before, doing one more sit-up, or playing with the grandchildren for a little while longer — a conscious development of accomplishment is being born. A permanent understanding through awareness of our shortcomings and our will to succeed as we go through the procedure of accomplishing something, achieving a goal, or reaching a start.

Accomplishment does not always mean that the goal has been attained. Maybe the swimming pool was just too long that last time around. Maybe rebounding took the breath from you a little sooner than you would have liked. But the accomplishment in the exercise is not just meeting the standard, but recognizing when you cannot and vowing to repeat it until you can. Success is not everything. Trying to be successful is the core of success. Never giving up, finding within yourself the determination to keep going, to push a little harder the next time and to walk away from a challenge knowing that you've given it your all. Then next time, the results may be different, because you will be back.

This philosophy applies to all of life's challenges, not just exercise.

Work requires a great deal of tenacity. When the report comes back with criticisms from the boss, the right attitude would be to approach it as a challenge to do better next time and not to view it as a personal failure. When your baby son does not tie his shoelaces on the first, second, fifteenth or thirty-fifth try, keep going back, be patient with him and yourself and, eventually, there will be a bow. When a relationship worth saving seems to be crumbling faster than you can pick up the pieces, determination and love, just as in exercise, will make the end result of emotional labors clear, and you will keep working until the goal is attained.

In the beginning, we look in the mirror and ask ourselves, can exercise really change all the mistakes I've made, physically and mentally? With commitment, yes it can. Gradually a more fit, fine-tuned body is born, and a better attitude grows right along with it. Maybe you're not going to become perfect, but you're going to be able to come forward.

Maybe you're not going to be ideal. But you're going to be able to cope, to do something, to act on, to move on, and to be.

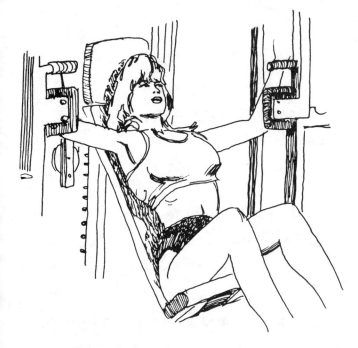

CHAPTER 12

The Consciousness of Creation: Our Power Through Exercise

Creation is a gift from a higher power: Someone larger than us Who looks down and keeps track of our accomplishments, our failures and our potential as a race of human beings. One of the most significant accomplishments we can have as human beings is to create as we have been created. And to recreate when what we have created is not meeting its fullest potential.

Through ingenuity, imagination and education, the human race has manufactured miraculous inventions that transport us realms above the next living creature. We do all of this with a blessing from above, because remember, this power of creation is a gift.

Man has created transcontinental flights that spirit us from Australia to England in a matter of hours. We can pick up a device called a telephone and exchange pleasantries with a friend thousands of miles away. We can travel as fast as 100 miles per hour in a machine made of steel and plastic called an automobile, and we can ferret information out of the darkest, largest tomb of a library within seconds through the technology of an index system in a molded box called a computer.

We have taken our ability to create, and changed the world. How we communicate, entertain, work and intereact has all been changed by our gift of creation. We have 100 percent support from the universe to create and recreate ourselves and our world.

So how can we blame someone else or something else when we become slouches, lazy, nonmoving creatures of habit stuck in front of a moving, idiotic box, wasting away into a death of toxic stillness? We can change that scenario by reinventing ourselves. It is called replication consciousness.

Replication consciousness is recognizing our ability to be aware of our state and change it. Consciousness is when we know we are sick, tired, listless, unhealthy, unhappy and bored. A change needs to be made, we say to ourselves. I cannot go on like this.

Replication is the rebuilding of that consciousness, which will expand the knowledge, thus the conversation will go something like: " I cannot go on like this and I can do something about it." Expanding the consciousness, or all things you are aware of, is a hard process. It is hard to deal with more than a few things at a time. Whatever is exactly in front of you is generally what you're dealing with.

Imagine if in the next minute someone bestowed on you the gift of ultimate, unlimited consciousness, meaning that you were capable of thinking all things there were to think. That notion is unfathomable. How could one person possibly think all the things that there are to think when we don't know all of the things?

But the very thought that you cannot think of all the things that you can think prevents you from the very thought. Did you follow that? Confusing, yes. Factual, yes. It's like trying to imagine the vastness of the universe past the Milky Way. Well, we are not sure yet what is past the Milky Way, so it is hard to imagine. But if you will not even think about imagining the universe past the Milky Way, then you have cut yourself off from even contemplating the thought.

Limited consciousness means limited creation. If you think, "I'm too old for this exercise" or "I'm too sick for this exercise" or "I'm too young for this exercise," then you have limited yourself before you have even considered the possibilities. Some people say to themselves before they even try, I can't walk two miles. I can't swim two laps. I can't do dance aerobics. They might have just as well stopped breathing because their life is over. Everything they will ever know, they have learned because they have prevented themselves from growing.

How about changing the negative "I can't" into a positive "I will"? Changing the body does not take years or decades, but sometimes changing the mind can take that long because people refuse to see beyond their experience and take that leap of faith in themselves. Anyone can change their body within six to nine months, but first you must have the consciousness of creation. A vision, a view of what you will look like when your life improves.

When you exericse, look at a magazine cover, at the beautiful people on the cover. Imagine you are them, full of confidence and self-assurance. You may not want to look like them. You should want **your** body to be the best it can be, not a clone of someone else's. That is the way to create. That is what people do to rid themselves of disease and find life again. They get that image of life and prosperity into their minds, and they do not let it go. Their life depends upon it.

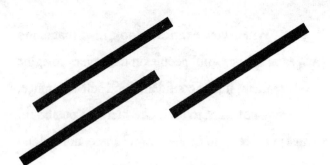

Final Note

Exercise is a whole, encompassing life element that supplements the mind, the body and the spirit. It cleans the body, uplifts it, energizes it and completes it. Exercise is a natural process of self-creation endorsed by the universe and heralded by every living creature that inhabits the Earth. It elongates the life, expands the mind, strengthens the muscles and breathes hope into a soul that has given up on its ability.

Exercise has the same characteristics as spirituality in that it has no bounds. Exercise can help us reshape our world, take us to new levels, and release us from previous bonds that were gaining strength as we sat umoving and still in a world that was passing us by.

As in spirituality, there is no way we can fully understand the power that comes through living well. As our bodies become less and less of a concern, our mind takes on new dimensions and responsibilities. Instead of worrying about weight because it is under control, we concentrate on how to make the world a better place or how did we as a human race come to be?

There is infinite potential in exercise. And it is part of our destiny to unlock that potential and use it to further the progress of the development of our hearts, minds and souls for happiness of our lives.

Bibliography

1. Freedman, Rita, Ph.D. *Bodylove: Learning to Like Our Looks — and Ourselves. A Practical Guide for Women.* Harper & Row Publishers, New York, 1988, p. 117.
2. *Bodylove*, p. 117.
3. Forsythe, Kenneth, M.D. and Feineman, Neil. *Athletics for Life; Optimal Fitness Through Recreational Sports.* Simon & Schuster, Inc., New York, 1985, p. 174.
4. *Athletics for Life*, p. 174-185.
5. *Athletics for Life*, p. 185.
6. Bailey, Overt. *The New Fit or Fat.* Houghton Mifflin Company, Boston, 1991, p. 30.
7. *Fit or Fat.* p. 30.
8. *Athletics for Life.* p. 45.
9. *Athletics for Life.* p. 77-78.
10. *Athletics for Life.* p. 131-133.
11. *Fit or Fat.* p. 79.
12. *Fit or Fat.* p. 83-91.
13. *Fit or Fat.* p. 110.
14. Prussin, Rebecca, M.D.; Harvey, Philip, Ph.D.; DiGeronimo, Theresa Foy. *Hooked on Exercise: How to Understand and Manage Exercise Addiction,* Simon & Schuster, Inc., New York, 1992. p. 129.
15. *Hooked on Exercise.* p. 22.
16. *Hooked on Exercise.* p. 94.

Hippocrates Health Insitute Offers an Unsurpassed Health Vacation

You are invited to attend our in-house guest program, which will teach you how to make exercise and healthful eating a part of your daily routine. For four decades people have been acquiring the needed education and motivation to change their inappropriate exercise and eating habits by spending this valuable time with us. Several weeks is the usual length of our program, but longer or shorter stays can be arranged. For more information you may call or write to our reservations clerk.

For those of you who desire involvement in the health field our Health Educator Course is considered by many in the field to be one of the most complete, state-of-the-art progressive health educations available anywhere. The pace is fast and the instructors are demanding, but the rewards more than compensate. Contact us for complete details regarding this eight-week health experience.

For four decades Hippocrates Health Institute has offered literature, tapes (audio and video), juicers and health equipment, along with whole food supplements, all of which are available to you with a call to the Institute.

Hippocrates Health Institute
1443 Palmdale Court
West Palm Beach, Florida 33411
(407) 471-8876

NOTES

NOTES